ALDARA

MW01269272

The Complete Guide

Effective Strategies for Managing Common Skin Conditions

Dr. Lillian Dermott

Contents

CHAPTER ONE

Overview of Aldara
(Imiquimod)

Aldara is another name for Imiquimod which is topical medication that can be applied on the skin in the treatment of several skin illnesses. Unlike conventional therapies that go straight to damaging the pathogens or any cells causing the disease, Aldara assists the immune system respond to the illness. This topical immune response modifier has an application in actinic keratosis, superficial basal cell carcinoma and genital warts. It is evident that Imiquimod functions through stimulating toll-like receptor 7 (TLR7) in cells and, later, cytokines, which work to improve the body's capability to detect and destroy improper cells and infections. This has put Aldara as an essential instrument in treatment of skin ailments that require immune-mediated therapy.

Mechanism of Action

It has effectively and safely treated various skin diseases that are prompted by the Immune system but Imiquimod does not work directly on any abnormal cells or pathogens. However, it escalates the body's natural immune response to infection and disease and so does not directly target HIV. Namely, Imiquimod acts selectively to toll-like receptor 7 (TLR7) on dendritic cells and other immune cells. This binding, in turn, relieves cytokines such as interferon-alpha, tumor necrosis factor-alpha and interleukin. The above cytokines are involved in initiating and regulating immune response mechanisms that enable a given body to recognize and destroy unusual cell formations, including skin cancers and warts.

Administration and Dosage

Patients and caregivers applying Aldara cream are usually advised to put the medication on the affected area as directed and leave it on for a certain amount of time prior to rinsing off. Apparently, the period of application as well as the frequency of application depends on ailment that is being treated. For instance, when used in the treatment of genital warts, Aldara is normally administered three times a week until the warts disappear or for a maximum of sixteen weeks. In the treatment of actinic keratosis, application is made on the skin twice in a week for 16 weeks. The dos and don'ts are quite essential to be followed by the patient as per the healthcare provider's advice to gain optimal benefits with the least side effects.

Primary Uses

Imiquimod commonly goes by the brand name Aldara, and it is

primarily applied to the skin to treat specific skin diseases by enhancing the immune system.

Actinic keratosis is a kind of precancerous skin disease which presents with rough, scaly skin changes on the parts of the body exposed to the sun- face, ears, neck, scalp, chest, back of the hands, forearms or lips. These patches are as a result of the cumulative effect of ultraviolet (UV) radiation from the sun.

In this instance, Aldara is administered topically two times a week for 16 weeks in order to rekindle the immune system's capability of identifying and eradicating the precancerous, or abnormal, existence. This assists in avoiding the advancement of actinic keratosis to squamous cell carcinoma.

Superficial basal cell carcinoma is also another skin cancer which originates from the basal cells in the epidermis of the skin. It is somehow less invasive and only stays at the outer layers of the skin.

In this case too, Aldara is used for the treatment of small individual superficial lesions of BCC mainly in situations where surgery is undesirable. It is normally used five times a week for six weeks, making it easy for patients to adhere to their recommended schedule. The immune response that is triggered by Imiquimod assists in the elimination of the cancerous cells.

Acquired Genital and Perianal Warts is a sexually transmitted disease resulting from the human papillomavirus (HPV) and manifest in the genital and perianal regions. They are communicable and may be accompanied by immense discomfort.

Again, in this case, Aldara is prescribed and administered three times weekly until the warts disappear, or for as long as 16 weeks. This particular cream operates on the fact that it helps to boost the local immunity around the affected area and this helps in clearing the viral infection and avoiding any future break out.

Administration and Dosage

Aldara is in the form of a topical solution that is applied directly to the affected skin area; this is done depending on the nature of the skin disease in terms of the time that is taken and the number of times that it is administered. Aldara for genital warts is regularly used thrice per week, until the warts disappear or up to a maximum of 16 weeks. For actinic keratosis, it is applied twice weekly for 16 weeks and for rosacea; it is also used, but the course may be different. Compliance to the particulars of care recommended by the healthcare provider is important since correct dosages give optimum results without side effects.

Alternatives to Aldara (Imiquimod)

Cryotherapy is considered one of the main rivals to Aldara and is based on the use of liquid nitrogen, which helps to freeze the regions with damaged skin cells. In clinical practice it is employed in the management of actinic keratosis, early basal cell carcinoma and certain types of viral warts. It is the most efficient type of treatment used for eradicating the certain lesions within the shortest time possible and with added positive outcomes. Despite being associated with pain, possibly needing several sessions, as well as causing blistering or pigmentary alteration.

Another significant option that is related to Aldara is 5-Fluorouracil. It is classified as a topical chemotherapy agent that has the ability of interfering with the synthesis of DNA among the fast-growing cells. In this country it is mostly prescribed for actinic keratosis, and superficial basal cell cancer.

Proven useful in management of precancerous and cancerous skin conditions, a widely used technique. It can also cause localized inflammation, erythema, vesicle and ulceration.

Apart from the aforementioned options among the remedies, Topical retinoids help in the acceleration of the cell's turnover rate and it also possesses an anti-cancer effect.

This is used in ointment form sometimes in the treatment of actinic keratosis and other precancerous skin diseases. Useful in treating precancerous lesions and soothes skin but may lead to skin rash, dryness and formation of a scaly layer on the skin.

Common Pitfalls Pertaining to the Use of Aldara (Imiquimod)

This section should comprise common pitfalls that may be encountered when using Aldara (Imiquimod).

Since side effects and the overall effectiveness of Imiquimod depends on certain parameters, precaution must be taken to ensure that Imiquimod is used in the right manner. Here are some common mistakes to avoid while using Aldara:

1. Using the cream more often or less often as talking to the doctor can cause severe skin reactions while low utilization can hamper the treatment process.

Therefore, the general recommended guidelines should be strictly complied to; the application should thus be done twice a week in the case of actinic keratosis, five times a week for superficial basal cell carcinoma and thrice a week for genital warts.

2. Side effects of excessive use include irritation of the skin at the point of application manifested by redness, itching and burning sensation.

Implement it lightly on the affected region according to the prescription of your doctor, or the dosage recommended by your healthcare provider.

3. It also has increased side effects, where clothing articles, bandages or dressings that help trap the cream on the skin help in the absorption of the drug. Occlusive dressings should not

be placed on the area treated with the agent unless your healthcare provider has advised to do so.

4. Failure to wash one's hands properly after applying the cream may lead to the spreading of the cream to other parts or to other people. Therefore, always make sure to wash your hands

with soap and warm water after the application of the cream.

5. To healthy, affected, or injured skin including cuts, chap or cracked areas the use of the product increases soreness and or worse reactions. It is always wise to try and use only on the areas that are affected as recommended by the doctor.

Should not be used on damaged, injured or infected skin.

Interactions of Aldara (Imiquimod)

Imiquimod seems to affect mainly the immune system and not directly associated drugs as the main type of interaction. Nevertheless, certain factors should be noted concerning interactions and possible impact.

Applying any other topical preparations with corticosteroids or other immunomodulating agents in the same treatment area as Aldara may decrease the effectiveness of Aldara, or at least increase the risk of skin reactions. Inform the patient not to apply any other topical medication or product on the same area as Aldara. These are creams that patients might use for fungal infection, bacterial infection, or sunburn that can interfere with Aldara's efficacy or increase the level of skin reactions.

As for the contraindications, the skin irritation worsened if it was under the influence of direct sunlight or UV light. This could cause skin reactions such as redness, burning or skin peeling at severe options which are not recommended.

Shelter treated parts from the sun and Ultra violet light. Find sunscreen that has a high SPF and put on a hat and other protective clothing to avoid getting excessively exposed to the sun rays.

Despite the lack of direct interactions with other systems, effects of other systemic immune system modulators or immunosuppressants might theoretically affect the implementation of Aldara on the immune response. You should also tell your doctor the following, any systemic medications that you are on, particularly immunosuppressive drugs. Now, your actual healthcare provider can decide whether there are any interactions or whether some doses have to be changed.

Also, Danes apply products with alcohol, astringents, or

other unpleasant compounds to the skin; in this case, they intensify skin irritation when using Aldara. Avoid rubbing the area gently and use products which are not harsh on the skin where the treatment will be done. Do not use products that may worsen the skin's condition and aggravate the problem.

When to Visit a Doctor

Internalization with your healthcare provider is recommended when using Aldara. Thus, awareness of severe or uncommon side effects and seeking help from a healthcare professional if such reactions are noticed can actually assist in controlling any potential complications and make the treatment more secure and efficient. If uncertain, always seek the advice of your doctor to avoid worsening the condition of the patient.

THE END

Made in the USA
Las Vegas, NV
13 September 2024

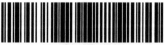

95156744R00022